EVERYTHING ABOUT FAT LOSS:

The ultimate no-nonsense manual

By

Jim K. Call

TABLE OF CONTENT

INTRODUCTION

Many times, the fat loss remains poorly understood. Have you ever wondered where the weight disappears when you lose it? If you're unsure, you're not by yourself. We'll go over the science of fat loss here. It will also include helpful weight-loss advice.

You may believe that fat can be converted into muscle or energy. However, it's not that easy. Let's examine the procedure in more detail. We'll examine fat's function. We'll look at how fat is burned by your body. We will discuss the variables that influence weight loss. Finally, we will discuss weight control advice.

Fat's function in the human body

Fat plays an important role. These are the following:

• Energy storage: Triglycerides found in fat store excess energy.

• Producing hormones: Fat tissue produces hormones that regulate numerous biological processes.

• Keeping us warm: Fat provides insulation.

Types of fat in the body

There are two primary categories of body fat:

White adipose tissue (WAT): It is an energy-storing organ. Fatty acids are released when it is low on energy. It is present around your organs and beneath your skin.

BAT, or brown adipose tissue, is considered "healthy" fat. It burns calories to regulate body temperature. It originates in the muscle. Compared to WAT, it contains more mitochondria.

How fat is stored and used by our body

Triglycerides and the process of storing energy

Overindulging in food turns excess energy into fat. Triglycerides are the form in which this fat is kept. Atoms of carbon, hydrogen, and oxygen are found in triglycerides. If you continue to eat too much, you will eventually put on weight. Additionally, your body composition varies.

The purpose of every kind of body fat

Body Fat Type and Function

White Adipose Tissue (WAT): synthesis of hormones, insulation, and energy storage

Adipose Brown Tissue (BAT) controls body temperature through heat-producing calorie burn

The Process of Burning Fat

Your body must turn to stored fat for energy to lose weight. Your fat cells shrink as a result of this. How then can we bring this about? Let's talk about the oxidation of fat.

Fat conversion to useful energy

Acidification and oxidation

The process known as lipolysis allows the circulation to contain accumulated triglycerides that are released from fat cells. They are converted into unbound fatty acids. Following that, these fatty acids undergo beta-oxidation, which releases carbon dioxide, water, and ATP (adenosine triphosphate) molecules. All of the body's cells get their energy from ATP.

Byproducts of fat loss and how the body excretes them

Carbon dioxide, water, and energy

Stored fat decomposes to produce energy, CO_2, and water.

Where Does Fat Go During the First Stages of Loss?

Patterns of body fat decrease

Individuals may experience varying patterns of fat loss. This is caused by a combination of genetics, sex, and lifestyle choices. But keep in mind that you cannot lose weight by targeting a single body component at a time.

Factors Influencing the Distribution of Fat Loss

Your body's composition, hormones, and genetics can all influence where and how you lose fat. Certain drugs and medical problems also may.

Stubborn Fat and the Difficulty of Losing It

Even though fat loss happens gradually, there could be harder spots. For example, the hips and tummy may prevent losing weight. Alpha 2-adrenergic receptors, which slow down fat burning, are more prevalent in them.

Chapter 1

Weight Loss Success: What Are the Key Strategies

maintaining a trim waist will help you live a longer life and look amazing. Increased risk of diabetes, cancer, and heart disease is associated with larger waistlines. Reducing weight—particularly adipose tissue—also enhances blood vessel health and elevates the quality of sleep. It is impossible to accurately target belly fat with diets. Overall weight loss, however, will help reduce your waistline; more significantly, it will help lower the harmful layer of visceral fat—a kind of fat found in the abdominal cavity that increases health risks despite being invisible to the naked eye.

Numerous weight-reduction regimens, fad diets, and outright scams all make the promise of rapid and simple weight loss. But maintaining a healthy, calorie-restricted diet along with more exercise still forms the cornerstone of effective weight loss. You need to permanently alter your lifestyle and health-related routines to lose weight successfully and sustainably.

How can those long-lasting adjustments be made? Think about implementing these six successful weight-loss strategies.

1. Ensure that you are prepared.

Time, effort, and a sustained commitment are necessary for long-term weight loss. Although you shouldn't give up on weight loss completely, you should be ready to make long-term changes to your eating and exercise routine. To assess your preparation, ask yourself the following questions:

Do I have the desire to shed pounds?

Are I being too sidetracked by other demands?

Do I turn to food as a stress reliever?

Are I ready to pick up new stress-reduction techniques or use existing ones?

Do I need more assistance from friends or professionals to handle my stress?

Am I ready to alter my eating patterns?

Will I be open to altering my exercise routine?

Do I have the time to devote to these modifications?

Consult your physician if you require assistance managing tensions or emotions that appear to be impediments to your preparedness. It will be simpler for you to make changes to your routines, stay engaged, and set goals when you're ready.

2. Discover your motivation

You cannot force someone else to lose weight. To pleasure yourself, you have to make dietary and activity adjustments. What can give you the overwhelming drive to stick to your weight loss plan?

To help you keep focused and motivated, write down your priorities, such as an impending trip or improved general health. Next, figure out how to ensure that, in times of temptation, you can access your motivating elements. For example, you may write a positive message to yourself and stick it on the refrigerator or pantry door.

For weight loss to be effective, you must accept responsibility for your actions, but having the appropriate kind of support is helpful. Choose allies who will uplift you rather than cause you any embarrassment, guilt, or harm.

Ideally, you should be surrounded by people who support you in your efforts to live a healthy lifestyle, who will also listen to your concerns and feelings, and who will spend time with you as you exercise or prepare wholesome meals. Accountability is another benefit that your support group can provide, and it can be a powerful incentive to maintain your weight-loss objectives.

If you would rather keep your weight-loss strategies a secret, hold yourself responsible by weighing in regularly, keeping a journal of your food and exercise regimen, or monitoring your progress with digital tools.

3. Make sensible objectives

Setting reasonable weight loss objectives can seem apparent. However, are you truly aware of what's practical? Overtime, aiming for a weekly weight loss of one to two pounds (0.5 to 1 kilogram). Generally speaking, you need to burn 500–1,000 more calories per day than you take in through regular physical activity and a reduced-calorie diet to lose 1–2 pounds per week.

At least as a starting point, 5% of your present weight might be a reasonable objective, depending on your weight. If you weigh 180 pounds (82 kilograms) is what you weigh, 9 pounds (4 kilograms). You can reduce your risk of developing long-term health issues like heart disease and type 2 diabetes by even losing this much weight.

Consider both process and outcome goals when you're creating your goals. "Take a 30-minute daily walk" is an illustration of a process objective. "Sheet 10 pounds" is an illustration of a result target. Although process goals are more important than end goals, since changing your habits is the key to weight loss, you should still set them.

4. Savor wholesome cuisine

Reducing your overall calorie consumption is a necessary part of embracing a new eating pattern that encourages weight loss. however, reducing calories doesn't have to mean giving up on flavor, satisfaction, or even meal prep convenience.

Eating more fruits, veggies, and whole grains that are plant-based is one approach to reducing your calorie intake. Aim for variety if you want to meet your goals without compromising taste or nutrients.

Start losing weight by using these suggestions:

Consume three servings of fruit and at least four servings of veggies each day.

Use whole grains instead of processed ones.

Make use of healthy fats in moderation, such as nuts, nut butter, avocados, olive oil, and vegetable oils.

Limit your intake of sugar to the least amount feasible, except for fruit's natural sugar.

Select lean meats and poultry in moderation, as well as low-fat dairy products.

5. Move and remain moving

while regular exercise and calorie restriction won't ensure weight loss on their own, they will offer you an advantage. exercise can help if food alone isn't enough to help you shed the excess calorie

Numerous other health advantages of exercise include elevating your mood, fortifying your heart, and lowering your blood pressure. Losing weight can be maintained with exercise as well. Research indicates that long-term weight reduction maintenance is associated with frequent physical exercise.

Your activity level, frequency, and duration all affect how many calories you burn. Regular aerobic activity, such as brisk walking, for at least 30 minutes most days of the week is one of the greatest strategies to shed body fat. For some people, this level of physical activity may not be enough to help them lose weight and keep it off.

Any additional exercise increases calorie burn. If you are unable to squeeze in formal exercise on any given day, consider ways you might improve your physical activity throughout the day. For instance, when shopping, park at the far end of the lot and make multiple journeys up and down the steps rather than taking the elevator.

6. Modify your viewpoint

If you want to successfully manage your weight over the long term, it takes more than just eating well and exercising for a few weeks or even months. These routines need to become second nature. Making honest assessments of your daily routine and eating habits is the first step in changing your lifestyle.

After assessing the particular challenges you have in your weight reduction journey, create a plan to gradually change the habits and perspectives that have thwarted your past efforts.

There will probably be sporadic setbacks. But after a failure, just get yourself up and try again the next day. Recall that you intend to make changes in your life. It will not occur in one go. The benefits of maintaining your healthy lifestyle will be worthwhile.

Chapter 2

Why is body fat significant?

The human body needs a healthy amount of body fat to function properly. Although having too much body fat has been associated with a higher risk of cancer, osteoarthritis, heart disease, and type 2 diabetes, having too little body fat can also be harmful.

Almost every cell in the body is made of fat; in fact, 60% of the brain is made of fat. Fat also provides energy to the body, much like protein and carbs do. In addition, hormones, body temperature, immunological response, reproduction, insulin signaling, and nutrition absorption are all influenced by fat. Furthermore, for the best absorption, body fat is necessary for the vital fat-soluble vitamins A, D, E, and K.

Men's and women's appropriate percentages of body fat

The precise body fat percentages for men and women that are associated with optimal health are still unknown, despite several decades of research and some broad guidelines.

Having said that, conventional criteria for men's body fat indicate that between 2% and 5% of body fat is needed, between 2% and 24% of body fat is deemed healthy, and over 25% of body fat is classified as obese. Women should aim for a body fat percentage of between 10% and 13%; between 10% and 31% is deemed healthy, while over 32% is categorized as obese. Stated differently, there exists a considerable spectrum of acceptability contingent upon an individual's gender and body shape.

Who Is Not Supposed to Try to Reduce Body Fat?

Unless specifically instructed otherwise by their physician, anyone who is immunocompromised, pregnant, nursing, malnourished, or dealing with a cancer diagnosis should not attempt to reduce their body fat. It is often advised in these situations that a trained medical expert be involved in the early stages of starting—or postponing—a weight reduction program.

Seniors should use caution as well. Sarcopenia is a specific type of obesity that affects the elderly in which there is an increase in fat mass and a loss in lean muscle mass. "You have to be extremely cautious when managing weight loss in elders because they require all muscle mass to stay functionally independent, and rapid weight loss might increase morbidity as well as death. This risk means that to preserve muscle mass during intentional weight loss, weight-bearing exercise must be included.

When is it OK to Try Losing body fat

Starting a body fat reduction program could be a good step toward better health if you don't fit into any of the above-mentioned prohibited groups and your body fat percentage is higher than the recommended range—especially if you also have excessive triglyceride and cholesterol levels.

Additionally, keep in mind that slower weight loss methods lead to a larger decrease in body fat percentage and fat mass than faster ones. It's generally safe to reduce total body fat by 0.5% per week or 2% per month. Depending on your initial weight, 1-2 pounds each week is a simpler way to measure it at home.

Furthermore, losing fat is not the same as losing weight overall. Body fat, lean muscle mass, organ weight, blood volume, and bone mass are all combined to give you the number you see on the scale. In actuality, you can gain more lean muscle and decrease fat without losing any weight. You are on the correct track if you notice that your waist is getting smaller but your total body weight stays the same.

How to decrease body fat

Fat loss that is both safe and effective takes time to achieve. Those who rapidly drop pounds by starving themselves, abstaining from food, or overdoing it at the gym typically end up gaining back all or most of the weight they originally lost. Results from weight loss will be fleeting if you don't keep your eyes on the broader picture." Are you prepared to reduce your body fat percentage for your well-being?

These are a dozen practical, research-backed strategies for losing weight:

1. Consume More Healthy Fats

Eat more healthful "good" fats, such as polyunsaturated fats, and restrict detrimental "bad" fats, such as trans fats, rather than following a low-fat diet.

Eat foods such as fish, avocados, olives and olive oil, eggs, nuts and nut butter, seeds, and dark chocolate to get heart-healthy monounsaturated and polyunsaturated fats. In the meanwhile, stay away from trans fats, which are present in processed snack foods, vegetable shortening, margarine, baked products, and fried foods.

2. Give Up Highly Processed Items and Refined Sugars

Ultra-processed foods (UPPs) make up over 70% of the average American diet starting at age 5, according to a recent study. This is bad news for body fat. In the modern Western diet, bread and baked goods, together with sauces, are the main sources of undesired oils and fats instead of meat and poultry. "UPPs are highly appetizing and addicting due to their high-fat content, which is often combined with added sweets and salt in an astonishing variety and quantity." Additionally, highly processed, low-nutrient, pre-packaged foods like cookies, doughnuts, chips, and margarine are frequently overindulged by people.

The average American consumes 152 pounds of refined sugar annually, which can significantly alter blood sugar regulation and raise insulin levels, both of which impact the storage of fat. Ultra-processed items often contain refined sugars, which are empty calories. "The body uses its fat reserves when calorie intake is reduced, which lowers the percentage of body fat."

3. Reconsider Your Drinking

Up to 30% of a person's daily caloric intake can be found in high-calorie sodas, alcohol, and other highly sweetened-liquids. These beverages frequently contain high-fructose corn syrup, which has been connected to fatty liver disease and other illnesses in humans.

Water consumption is crucial for burning fat that has been stored as well as fat from food and drink. Studies have shown that drinking more water increases lipolysis, or the breakdown of fat, and decreases the formation of new fat.

What volume of water is required? Drink half your body weight in ounces each day as a general guideline. In other words, aim to drink 75 ounces of water a day if you weigh 150 pounds.

4. Increase Protein

Rich protein diets can aid in weight loss by encouraging satiation—the sensation of fullness—maintaining muscle mass while reducing body fat, and boosting diet-induced thermogenesis—the process of burning calories during digestion.

Consuming protein also aids in lowering ghrelin production, which may help you crave fewer carbohydrates and sweets. According to one study, consuming 25% more protein than one would normally consume each day helped lower cravings by 60%, including those for late-night snacks. Increasing the amount of protein in your diet may also help your body burn more calories throughout the day by increasing metabolism.

Depending on your age, sex, and degree of exercise, try to get 15% to 25% of your daily calories from high-quality protein sources to aid in weight reduction.

5. Look for More Fiber

Compared to sugars, proteins, and carbs, fiber makes you feel fuller and takes longer to digest. According to research, dieters who followed a diet consisting solely of 30 grams of fiber per day experienced a notable weight reduction. in addition to aiding in weight loss, fiber also strengthens the heart, and the intestines, and reduces the risk of diabetes and some cancers. Dietary sources such as wheat bran, legumes, fruits, and oats are recommended by me.

Additionally, studies show that fiber effectively reduces stubborn belly fat, which is significant because having too much belly fat increases the risk of type 2 diabetes and cardiovascular disease, among other health problems.

6. Add Vinegar and Ferment as Supplements

One of the most important factors in safely reducing and maintaining body fat is a healthy gut microbiota. Consuming foods that are naturally fermented, such as yogurt, kimchi, pickles, sauerkraut, and kefir, provides the gut with beneficial bacteria and the substrates they require to flourish.

7. Throw Away Chemicals That Cause Fat

Even though you might not give it much thought, look for obesogens in your plastic if losing weight is your main concern.

Obesogens are covert substances that cause hormonal imbalances, seize control of our metabolic processes, and even promote the body's accumulation of fat. Reduced growth hormone secretion, abnormal cortisol levels, and increased insulin resistance can all result from exposure.

These chemicals that cause fat are present in food containers, plastics, herbicides, pesticides, artificial sweeteners, hormones injected into cattle, and non-stick cookware. Bisphenol-A (BPA), a synthetic estrogen used to harden plastic for products like water bottles and plastic food containers, is one type of obesogen you may be familiar with.

8. Incorporate Strength Training

Diet and exercise are equally crucial for fat loss. Additionally, lifting weights is a good idea if you want to maximize fat reduction.

Studies regularly demonstrate that when diet and resistance exercise are combined, the greatest reductions in fat mass occur. This is especially true when comparing diet alone with diet plus exercise. You'll also appear toned much quicker if you increase your lean muscle mass while decreasing your fat mass.

Consider seeking professional advice from a personal trainer if this is your first time incorporating resistance training into your fitness regimen. In the meantime, the Centers for Disease Control and Prevention (CDC) recommends that individuals engage in strength-training exercises at least twice a week that target all major muscle groups, including the arms, shoulders, back, legs, and hips.

9. Increase Heart Rate

Cardiovascular exercises, such as jogging, cycling, and walking for extended periods, are also crucial for fat loss. They increase metabolism and aid in effective calorie burning for both of you.

To maximize your fat-burning cardio routines, deduct your age from 220 to find your maximal heart rate. It appears that a heart rate between 70% and 80% of that range is the most efficient for burning fat. Additionally, the ideal quantity of cardio for fat loss will differ from person to person, just like many of the other factors discussed here. However, according to general CDC guidelines, one should engage in moderate-intensity aerobic activity for at least 150 minutes per week.

You should think about incorporating high-intensity interval training (HIIT) into your cardio routine if you want to accelerate your fat reduction. Short bursts of high-intensity exercise are interspersed with rest periods or lower-intensity workouts in high-intensity interval training (HIIT). Research indicates that this type of exercise can lead to an overall reduction in body fat of 28.5% more than steady-state aerobic exercises like power walking.

10. Raise Your NEAT

Non-workout activity The term thermogenesis, also known as NEAT, refers to all the calories you burn performing regular daily activities like cooking, cleaning, taking out the garbage, playing the piano, fidgeting, and so forth. Even while this exercise might not seem like much, every little bit helps in the fight against body fat.

Conversely, leading a sedentary lifestyle or spending excessive amounts of time sitting down might lead to an increase in body fat. In actuality, research indicates that obesity and poor NEAT are related. However, you risk losing it if you relocate it. Take the stairs, park your car at the far end of the lot, or help your neighbor bring their groceries inside as small adjustments you can do every day to fit in extra exercise.

11. Get More Sleep

Adults who sleep fewer than seven hours in 24 hours are more likely to be obese than those who consistently receive at least seven hours of sleep, according to research.

Getting enough sleep is crucial for building muscle and reducing weight. Lack of sleep affects the hormones that control hunger, ghrelin, and leptin, increasing the likelihood that you may engage in unhealthy eating behaviors.

Another hormone that increases when you don't get enough sleep is cortisol. It is also released by the body in reaction to stress and has a significant role in the build-up of fat in the abdominal region.

Feel free to use your desire to reduce your body fat percentage as an excuse to go to bed earlier, given the average adult only gets six hours of sleep or less. Sleeping your pounds away is the simplest approach to reducing weight.

12. Eat Slowly

"The average person's gastrointestinal tract takes around 20 minutes to begin alerting the brain when it is full. You may prevent unintentional overeating by giving your stomach the time it needs to alert your brain when you've had enough food by taking your time, slowing down, and savoring each bite as you go.

Eat until you're around 80% full, and then wait for your brain to process the food. Waiting a few minutes is likely to result in you eating less and reducing body fat before it builds up.

CHAPTER 3

The impact of your food environment

Personal aspects including taste preferences, emotional states, and hunger levels impact the foods we choose to eat. Our physical surroundings, which include the stores in our communities, the foods they sell, and their prices, as well as other, more indirect influences like our exposure to advertising and the government policies that shape the food system, also have an impact on them. Our social circles, which include our friends and family, also play a role. The term "food environment" refers to these and additional environmental factors.

Personal Factors

Personal characteristics including knowledge, taste preferences, emotional situations, and hunger affect the foods we choose to eat.

Research indicates that those with greater dietary knowledge typically make better decisions. However, knowledge on its own cannot solve bad eating habits. People can only resist handy, enticing meals for so long, especially when they're hungry, anxious, or exhausted. This is true even when they are actively attempting to make good choices.

What people consume is also greatly influenced by their priorities. According to surveys, when Americans are choosing foods, they put flavor, affordability, nutrition, and convenience in that order. Additionally, a lot of customers base their food choices on their values, giving public health, environmental stewardship, social justice, or animal welfare, for example, top priority. Customers may be more likely to "vote with their forks" in support of agricultural methods that suit their goals as they become more knowledgeable about these concerns.

Taste is a combination of smell, texture, and taste, as is commonly assumed. Sweet foods are naturally palatable to children, and dishes that combine sugar and fat are frequently very enticing. However, based on their experiences, people may and do learn to appreciate different tastes, and if they are exposed to a flavor frequently, they may grow to like it more. Our mothers' pregnancies also influenced our taste preferences even while we were still in the womb.

Social Factors

Our eating choices are influenced, for better or worse, by the individuals we spend time with.

According to research, people imitate the eating habits of their family, friends, and coworkers. Children were more likely to eat fruits and vegetables regularly in households where the parents did. According to the same theory, youngsters drank more soft drinks in homes where the parents drank more often. Adults in a different study were more inclined to eat more fruits and vegetables if they had

more acquaintances or colleagues who consumed five servings or more of fruits and vegetables daily.

When it comes to encouraging better eating habits, positive reinforcement often gets along well with both adults and children. According to studies, parental attempts to restrict what their kids eat—like denying them access to sweets—usually end up backfiring. It was more common for kids in these settings to want "limited" items and detest the nutritious foods they were made to eat under duress. On the other hand, research indicates that when parents provide explicit instructions while providing their kids the liberty to select healthful options, their eating habits tend to improve.

Food Stores

While candy, soda, and other items high in fat are readily available on street corners in many communities, many American households struggle to afford nutritious food. Compared to mostly-white or higher-income communities, low-income neighborhoods and communities of color, in particular, typically feature more fast food restaurants, convenience stores, and fewer supermarkets. What effects do these patterns have on the dietary habits and general health of the residents of such communities?

Researchers can survey retailers to determine if they sell fresh vegetables, for example, to gauge the availability of healthful food in a community. Supermarkets typically provide the greatest selection of healthful products at the most affordable costs when compared to smaller retailers. Notwithstanding these benefits, studies indicate that having a supermarket nearby does not always translate into a healthier diet. Other interventions could be used to urge people to shop and eat healthier. Examples of these include providing cooking demos and promotional discounts on fruits and vegetables.

Supermarkets may be a part of the answer, but distributing them to areas that lack them—like impoverished metropolitan areas—can be difficult. Supermarkets need a large amount of land, and urban land is frequently expensive and scarce. Store owners may believe they won't receive enough revenue from lower-class customers due to their claimed security worries.

People eat the foods they do for a variety of intricate reasons. Having access to a car, public transportation, or simply walkways could be the difference between grocery shopping and takeaway. Communities are attempting to increase access to healthy food in a variety of ways, such as:

• Increasing the amount of fruits and vegetables that small grocery stores and corner stores stock,

• Ensuring the usage of public benefits at farmers' markets, such as food stamps, and

Enhancing public transportation lines to grocery stores

Eateries

Roughly one-third of the calories consumed by most people come from meals served in cafeterias, restaurants, and other non-home environments. In just three decades, the percentage of calories from fast food outlets has surged considerably, rising from 3 to 13 percent. Nowadays, 30% of American children are thought to consume fast food establishments every day. Why should we be concerned about these trends?

Studies indicate that those who eat a greater proportion of their meals at restaurants tend to consume higher amounts of fat, calories, and less fruit, vegetables, and fiber. Additionally, they can be more susceptible to obesity and weight increase. Fast food restaurants added the most saturated fat and the least amount of fiber to American diets between 2005 and 2008; full-service restaurants added the most salt, while home-cooked meals were the healthiest on all three measures.

Additionally, restaurants frequently serve portions that are two to eight times bigger than those recommended by dietary guidelines.

For example, several fast-food businesses today serve hamburgers, French fries, and sodas in servings that are two to six times greater than they were when they were initially introduced. It has been demonstrated that larger serving sizes significantly increase customers' intake, frequently without their knowledge.

Customers frequently greatly underestimate the number of calories in meals and may not be aware of the fat and salt content of restaurant food.

School Cuisine

School cafeterias have often served as a battlefield between conflicting interests. The diets and health of young people in America are at risk because they spend more than one-third of their daily calories in school on average.

The majority of public and private schools provide lunches via the School Breakfast Program, the National School Lunch Program (NSLP), or both. According to research, kids who take part in federal meal programs tend to eat less sweetened beverages, sweets, and snacks and more fruits, vegetables, and dairy products. Nearly 60% of children enrolled in school meal programs come from low-income households, making the free and reduced-price meals provided through federal programs an essential defense against hunger.

Restrictions were placed in place by lawmakers when the NSLP was first implemented in 1946 to prevent private food manufacturers from entering schools. But by the 1970s, many school meal programs were underfunded, and private companies could provide meals effectively and affordably. As a result, they feared that "corporations [would] sell anything to the child as long as he has the money to pay for it." Wanting to preserve the nutritional quality of school meals. The lifting of restrictions allowed private vendors, including fast food chains and soft drink producers, to provide their goods—referred to as "competitive foods"—in schools.

Competitive meals may help schools raise much-needed funds, but there has long been a public health issue with the easy access to sugary drinks and high-fat, salty snacks in classrooms. However, it is anticipated that the kinds of competitive meals that are permitted to be offered at schools would alter.

Your Environment Affects What You Eat in Five Ways

Understanding your surroundings is a crucial first step if you're attempting to identify every aspect of your life that affects the decisions you make regarding the meals you eat.

It's simple to give in to influences that appear uncontrollable when attempting to form good eating habits.

Your choices are greatly influenced by the places you eat, the items you choose to put on your plate, the people you spend time with, the stores where you purchase food, and how your society presents food to you.

Therefore, it is your responsibility to manage your health. You can gain a significant advantage in the battle for improved nutrition by recognizing the factors that influence your decisions.

Here are five ways that your environment affects the foods you eat, along with some advice on how to maintain your health despite your circumstances.

Where You Eat

These days, unhealthy meals are readily available everywhere. Food is served in petrol stations, at sporting events, at your school or workplace, in the park where you work out, and pretty much wherever else you go.

You might be more inclined to give in to these persistent cravings and indulge in some of these items. Furthermore, the food offered at these establishments is probably not the healthiest.

Similar to fast food restaurants, convenience stores are particularly guilty when it comes to offering processed meals.

You might be more inclined to settle for a quick hamburger or burrito rather than looking for a healthier option if you work or attend school in a place where there aren't many other options.

If the setting in which you eat supports it, you can continue to stick your fork in your mouth even though you don't feel like eating or enjoying the food that is being provided. Techniques for reducing food intake in unhealthier settings include:

In a restaurant, ordering a salad is eighty percent more likely when you are seated by a window.

If you sit close to the bar, you have a 73% higher chance of ordering dessert.

Your eating habits might be altered by the location of your food in the kitchen. You can be tricking yourself into thinking that unhealthy meals are more important than healthier ones if you keep them in the areas of your kitchen that are most accessible and out of the way.

Additionally, studies revealed that the likelihood of eating the first item one sees is three times higher than that of eating the fifth.

How You Consume

How about the eating utensils you use?

You most likely only consider your fork to be a tool for shoving food in your mouth, but is there a chance that its size has an impact on how much you eat?

Compared to patrons using regular-sized forks, those using forks that were 20% larger than usual consumed less food overall and left more food on their plates.

One possible reason for this could be that those who use smaller forks feel as though they aren't satisfying their hunger sufficiently because they are getting less from each bite.

According to a Georgia Institute of Technology study, individuals who ate their ice cream from a larger bowl would have consumed 31% less. According to the same study, people consume roughly 92% of what they serve themselves.

You are more likely to eat more if you serve yourself more of anything!

The rise in portion sizes over the past few decades is another factor contributing to this issue. The same foods that people ate thirty years ago are now available in greater portions and with lower nutritional value, making it more difficult than ever for people to lose weight.

By being aware of serving quantities and educating yourself, you can take charge. Make sure you know how much a serving amount of cereal is before reaching into your cupboards for one. A full bowl might be closer to three servings than one, despite popular belief.

With your meal, you can request a to-go box and put only the food on your plate that you intend to consume, putting the remainder away for later.

With Whom You Eat

What you decide to put on your plate and put in your mouth might be greatly influenced by the individuals you share meals with. According to the Harvard School of Public Health, a lot of your adult dietary habits are influenced by the foods your family of origin served you growing up.

Depending on your ancestry, you might like foods that are representative of your culture. Even if they can taste good, meals from your heritage aren't necessarily the healthiest options available.

What you eat will not only be influenced by your ingrained subconscious prejudices toward particular foods but also by the people you eat with.

Social pressure can be really powerful, and you may be giving in to it without even realizing it, especially when you're among your peers in a relaxed setting.

According to a different study, you will start gaining weight once your peers do.

Even something as basic as what your pals choose to eat might have an impact on you. Even though you may have arrived at the dinner with the best of intentions—eating light and healthfully—you start to lose caution as soon as you hear what everyone else is eating.

Planning for meals is the greatest approach to combat these forces. Plan your meals ahead of time and abide by them. Decide not to be influenced by your friends' eating choices, even if it means putting in some effort.

Always be mindful of the potent influence of peer pressure, or as mindful as you can be. You don't have to do as your buddies do when you watch them idly reaching for a handful of chips. Resolve to resist the urge to participate in the casual dining trend of groupthink.

You can also prepare your meal ahead of time or place your order first. You should pack your food or get a short bite to eat in advance if you'll be attending a party where the food options might be restricted to the unhealthy dishes made by the hosts.

The Media And Advertising

As previously stated, a person's dietary choices are greatly influenced by their cultural background. However, because ingenious advertising permeates every aspect of our culture, we could be convinced to purchase goods we might not have needed otherwise.

In many respects, advertising is pretty brilliant. Sometimes we mock commercials, asking ourselves how anyone could fall for them.

However, the advertisements do more than merely persuade you to purchase the item. They often depict pleasant, smiling people using their stuff, giving you the impression that the product is positive. This is known by psychologists as emotional conditioning.

The emotional component of the brain is frequently targeted by news and advertising, which is why you may feel compelled to try a new product after hearing someone on television discuss it.

Just the packaging of food can have a significant influence on our purchasing decisions. Unhealthy meals are frequently exhibited in vivid colors with captivating graphics, whereas healthy, organic foods come in simpler, more affordable packaging.

A cognitive bias known as the "halo effect" leads us to believe that a product is superior to others just because our view of it has been slightly skewed.

Because marketers are well aware of this impact and take advantage of it, products with bold health claims on their packaging may persuade you to purchase one over the identical product that is sitting next to it without those phrases.

The supermarket

Purchase Wisely

Food stores have gotten quite good at quietly persuading you to buy the things they want you to buy.

Large shopping carts, as opposed to little baskets, might encourage you to load up on products so that your lone box of granola bars doesn't feel so empty.

Eggs, milk, and bread are the staple commodities that customers most frequently need in grocery shops, and they are arranged for optimal impact.

Fresh meats and baked items are usually arranged closer to the front, where their delicious fragrances will hit your senses, making you feel better and somewhat more hungry.

Since milk and eggs are frequently positioned closer to the back corners of stores, you will need to go past a plethora of other temptations to get to them.

The cheaper (and occasionally healthier) foods are positioned lower down or at the end of aisles where you have to search for them; name-brand items are typically positioned on middle and upper shelves where they are more likely to catch attention.

Avoid falling for their ploys! Make a list of everything you need before you head to the grocery store, and stick to it. Purchase only what you require to prepare wholesome meals.

CHAPTER 4

Portion Sizes

What does a portion size mean?

The recommended amount of each food item to be consumed during a meal or snack is known as the serving size. The quantity of food that you eat is called a portion. You risk consuming too few or too many of the nutrients you require if you consume more or less than the suggested serving amount.

A higher number of people than ever are unable to manage their weight, which is contributing to the obesity pandemic.

It is believed that larger portion sizes play a role in overindulging and unintended weight gain. According to research, a variety of things can affect how much you eat.

Nearly all that is served to them is usually consumed by the individual. Consequently, limiting portion sizes can aid in avoiding overindulging. Here are nine pointers for measuring and managing portion sizes when you're at home or on the go:

1. Make Use of Smaller Dinnerware

Research indicates that an individual's unconscious food intake can be influenced by the size of their glasses, plates, and spoons. Using huge dishes, for instance, might make food appear smaller, which frequently encourages overeating.

Those who used a large bowl ate 77% more spaghetti than those who used a medium-sized bowl in one research.

In another study, when offered bigger bowls and larger serving spoons, nutrition experts fed themselves 31% and 14.5% more ice cream, respectively.

It's interesting to note that the majority of individuals who consumed larger portions did not even realize their portion sizes had changed.

Therefore, you can cut down on the serving size and avoid overindulging by using a smaller plate, bowl, or serving spoon instead of your typical one. When they eat from a smaller plate, most individuals feel just as full as when they eat from a larger one.

2. Make a portion guideline using your plate

If you find it difficult to weigh or measure your meal, consider using your plate or bowl as a guide for portion control.

You may use this to figure out what the ideal macronutrient ratio is for a well-balanced meal.

For each meal, here's a general guide:

Salad or veggies: half a plate

Superior grade protein Meat, chicken, fish, eggs, dairy, tofu, beans, and pulses make up a quarter of a meal.

Complex carbohydrates: Starchy vegetables and whole grains make up a quarter of a dish.

foods heavy in fat: Half a tablespoon (7 grams) - comprising butter, oils, and cheese

Keep in mind that since everyone's nutritional demands are different, this is only a general guide. For instance, those who engage in more physical activity frequently need to eat more.

Filling up on veggies and salads will help you avoid overindulging in calorie-dense foods because they are inherently low in calories but high in fiber and other nutrients.

Certain manufacturers supply portion-control plates if you would like more advice.

3. Use Your Hands to Guide the Serving

Using your hands is another method of determining the right portion size without the need for any measurement equipment.

Larger persons who need more food generally have larger hands since your hands normally match your body size.

For each meal, here's a general guide:

High-protein foods include meat, fish, chicken, and beans; for women, one palm-sized serving, and males, two palm-sized portions.

salads and vegetables: A part the size of a fist for women and two portions the size of a fist for men

High-carb foods: Whole grains and starchy vegetables, one cupped-hand serving for women and two for men.

foods heavy in fat: For example, one thumb-sized piece of butter, oils, and nuts for women, and two for men.

When dining out, request a half portion.

Large portions are a common occurrence in restaurants.

In actuality, restaurant serving sizes can be up to eight times bigger than normal serving sizes, with an average increase of roughly 2.5 times.

You can always request a children's meal or a half quantity when dining out.

You'll cut down on calories and avoid overindulging by doing this.

Instead of ordering a main course, you might have an appetizer and a side dish or split the dinner with someone.

Additional recommendations include requesting that sauces and dressings be served separately, getting a side salad or vegetables, and staying away from all-you-can-eat buffet buffets where it's simple to overindulge.

5. Have a Glass of Water Before Every Meal

Partition control will naturally be aided by drinking a glass of water up to 30 minutes before a meal.

Drinking lots of water will help you feel less peckish. You can tell the difference between hunger and thirst when you're properly hydrated.

Drinking 17 ounces (500 ml) of water before each meal led to a 44% higher loss in weight over 12 weeks in one research of middle-aged and older adults, most likely because they consumed less food.

Similarly, older persons who were overweight or obese and drank 17 ounces (500 ml) of water half an hour before eating consumed 13% fewer calories without making an effort to alter.

In another study, young men of normal weight who drank the same amount of water right before a meal reported feeling fuller and eating less.

As a result, drinking a glass of water before every meal can promote portion control and help avoid overindulging.

6. Proceed Gradually

Eating rapidly reduces your awareness of fullness, which raises the risk of overindulging.

Slowing down will help you consume less food overall because it can take your brain up to 20 minutes to recognize when you're full after eating.

For instance, eating slowly was associated with higher feelings of fullness and lower food consumption than eating quickly in a study of healthy women.

Moreover, the ladies who ate gradually seemed to take greater pleasure in their food.

Furthermore, eating when occupied, on the road, or while watching TV increases the risk of overeating.

As a result, the likelihood that you will enjoy your meal and manage your portion sizes rises when you concentrate on it and refuse to rush.

It is advised by medical professionals to take smaller bites and to chew each mouthful at least five or six times before swallowing.

7. Avoid Eating Right Out of the Container

Food served in huge containers or packaged in jumbo proportions tends to promote overindulgence and reduces awareness of serving amounts.

This particularly applies to snacks.

Research indicates that regardless of the flavor or quality of the food, consumers often eat more out of large packages than tiny ones.

For instance, when candy was provided from a large container as opposed to a tiny one, consumers ate 129% more of it.

8. Recognize the Proper Serving Size

Studies show that we can't always trust our instincts about the right amount to eat. This is due to the wide range of influences on portion control.

Nonetheless, to accurately measure your consumption and weigh meals, it can be beneficial to get a scale or measuring cup.

Proper portion knowledge is also increased by reading food labels.

Moderation of intake can be achieved by being aware of suggested serving sizes for regularly consumed items. Here are a few instances:

One-half cup (75 or 100 grams) of cooked pasta or rice

Salad and veggies: 1-2 cups (150-300 grams)

Cereal for breakfast 40 grams, or one cup

One-half cup (90 grams) of cooked beans

Two tablespoons (16 grams) of nut butter

Three ounces (85 grams) of cooked meats

It's not necessary to measure your food every time. But for a brief while, doing so might help you become conscious of what constitutes a suitable portion size. You might not need to measure everything after a while.

In another study, participants who received snacks in 100-gram snack packs as opposed to standard-sized packets consumed more than 180 fewer grams of snacks weekly.

To avoid consuming more snacks than necessary, remove the snacks from their original box and place them into a small bowl.

The same holds for large servings of family meals. Before serving, report the food onto plates rather than serving it straight off the stove. By doing this, you can avoid piling food on your plate and deter others from asking for seconds.

9. Keep a Nutrition Journal

According to research, people are frequently taken aback by how much food they consume.

According to one study, 21% of those who said they had eaten more because their serving bowls were bigger said they had not.

You may become more conscious of the kinds and quantities of food you're eating by keeping a journal of everything you eat and drink.

Those who kept a food journal during weight reduction studies generally lost more weight.

This most likely happened as a result of their diet being modified in response to their increased awareness of what they were eating, especially their poor choices.

How does one distinguish between a serving and a portion?

A portion is the amount of food you decide to have in one sitting, whether it's at home, in a restaurant, or out of a box. A portion or portion size the amount of food specified on a product's Nutrition Facts or food label is an external link.

Serving sizes vary throughout different items. Sizes can be expressed as numbers, such as three crackers, pieces, slices, ounces, grams, or cups. The amount you choose to eat will determine whether or not your portion size fits the serving size.

On the label, the number of servings is indicated at the top. Serving size is listed directly above "Servings per container." A cup is the serving size for frozen lasagna in the example below. The container, however, holds four servings. You would be consuming two servings if you wanted to consume two cups or half of the package.

To determine how many calories you would be getting, do some math.

280 calories in 1 serving.

$280 \times 2 = 560$ calories from 2 servings

Eating two servings in this instance would result in consuming twice as many calories and other nutrients as specified on the food label.

In what ways have suggested serving sizes evolved?

The Food and Drug Administration (FDA) of the United States modified the serving sizes of several foods and beverages so that the amounts on the labels more closely matched our daily consumption. Certain serving sizes on food labels may be greater or smaller than they were previously due to recent changes made to the Nutrition Facts label (see Figure 2 below). For example, half a cup used to be the serving size for ice cream. It is now two and a third cups. Yogurt used to come in 8-ounce portions. It weighs six ounces now.

Recall that the serving size listed on a label does not indicate the amount of food or liquids you should consume.

What is the recommended serving size?

A food's serving size may be greater or lower than the recommended quantity to consume. This is because the number of calories you require daily to either maintain or reduce your weight may vary depending on your age, height, present weight, and metabolism.

what gender you are and how active you are

For instance, a 150-pound woman whose primary form of exercise is a quick stroll once a week will require fewer calories than a woman of the same size who participates in strenuous exercise, like running, many times a week.

Check out the following tools to determine how many calories are just right for you.

Based on your age, sex, and degree of physical activity, the Dietary Guidelines for Americans, 2020–2025 might help you estimate how many calories you would require each day.

You can create your own calorie and exercise plans using the Body Weight Planner tool to help you reach and stay at your target weight.

How can I benefit from the Nutrition Facts label on food?

The majority of packaged foods have the FDA's Nutrition Facts label printed on them. You can find out how many calories, fat, protein, carbs, and other nutrients are in a portion of food by reading the label. A lot of packaged goods come in multiple servings. The calorie count in one serving size is now listed on the redesigned product label in larger text than before, making it simpler to read.

Extra useful information on the product label

Other helpful details regarding what's in a single food portion are included on the product label, like:

• Total fat.

• Sugar additions. As per the 2020–2025 Dietary Guidelines for Americans, added sugars should make up no more than 10% of your daily caloric intake.

According to the Dietary Guidelines for Americans, 2020–2025, a person should consume no more than 2,300 mg of sodium daily, or even less for children under the age of 14.

additional nutrition. Americans frequently don't get enough potassium and vitamin D. For this reason, serving guidelines for each of these nutrients are included on the revised product label shown in Figure 3. Vitamins A and C are no longer included on food labels because the majority of Americans obtain adequate of them in their diets. But food producers are free to add them if they so want.

The significance of serving sizes

• Easily digest food;

• Achieve and sustain a healthy weight

It is typically not advised for cancer patients undergoing active treatment to try to lose weight at this time. Before making any dietary changes, consult a qualified dietician or your healthcare team.

- Maintaining energy levels throughout the day.
- managing blood sugar levels.
- money back in your pocket.

Chapter 5

Weight stigma

What is the stigma associated with weight?

Weight stigma is defined as "the discriminating acts and attitudes geared towards persons because of their size and weight" by the World Obesity Federation.

Discrimination based on weight occurs to older persons daily in retail establishments, dining establishments, public transit, job, and healthcare environments. Relationships within the family are impacted by weight stigma. In fact, "fat shaming" is so pervasive in contemporary culture that many may be blind to its existence. Furthermore, research indicates that weight discrimination is on the rise in tandem with rising obesity rates.

Regrettably, prejudice towards those who are obese remains socially acceptable in North America. This leaves a sizable portion of the populace defenseless against obviously unfair treatment and without many options for assistance and protection. As of right now, discrimination based on weight is not prohibited by any federal laws. Consequently, it is rare to question or challenge this kind of behavior. In actuality, it's frequently disregarded.

Which instances of weight stigma are there?

People who struggle with weight are often misunderstood. Among them could be assumptions and generalizations like:

• Obesity patients are careless and lethargic men and women. They are weak in self-control and determination.

• People bear extra weight as a result of decisions they've made; their struggles are "their fault."

• A bigger body size is unpleasant and unsightly.

Overweight people are assumed to be less intelligent; obese people maintain poor hygiene; and those who are obese have lower chances of success.

Because the media frequently promotes a slender body as the ideal, stigmatization of those who are obese is widely maintained. People who are overweight are notably underrepresented in advertisements, motion pictures, and television programs, especially women. They are frequently depicted as objects of mockery or inferiority when they do appear on screen—the witty sidekick in place of the hero, or the astute best friend in place of the romantic interest. In contrast to performers with obesity, who are regarded as unpopular, belligerent, or rude, slim-figured stars are portrayed as successful and well-liked.

In their everyday lives, older persons encounter more subdued manifestations of weight stigma. For instance, many doctor's clinics lack examination tables and gowns large enough to fit individuals of greater stature. A person who is quite overweight will not be able to fit into most seats on commercial aircraft. In this instance, purchasing two seats is frequently necessary for the traveler to sit comfortably during the journey.

What negative effects does weight stigma have?

Weight stigma can have detrimental social, psychological, and bodily impacts, including the following, according to the Obesity Action Coalition (OAC):

• Negative body image and low self-esteem

• Lowered income and less opportunities for advancement at work; depression and worry; rejection from family and friends; poor quality of personal connections;

• Sedentary or exercise avoidance behaviors; • Adverse weight control practices (such as eating disorders)

Contrary to what one might think, weight discrimination does not encourage people to lose weight. According to research, fat shaming and anti-obesity bias may be the cause of weight increase. This is because stress, which is a result of being exposed to weight bias, impairs self-control and encourages binge eating. In one study, individuals who experienced a significant degree of internalization of weight bias were found to be three times more likely than non-internalized individuals to be at risk of heart disease and diabetes due to metabolic syndrome, which is a cluster of three out of four health conditions including elevated blood sugar, high blood pressure, high body mass index, and high cholesterol.

Obesity can also make it difficult to access high-quality medical treatment. Obesity patients receive less time from some primary care physicians because they perceive them as "non-compliant." A provider's ability to provide high-quality care may be compromised by bias against patients who struggle with weight concerns. Perceived discrimination by providers may also discourage obese individuals from seeking medical attention for health issues.

What strategies may be used to combat the stigma associated with obesity?

It will take time and work to pass legislation outlawing discrimination based on weight and to alter deeply ingrained societal attitudes around obesity. Nonetheless, there are actions you can take right now to combat weight stigma if you're an obese older adult:

• Inform other people. Many folks, whether they be friends or relatives, just don't know enough about obesity. Dispel popular myths by describing obesity as a long-term medical illness with a wide range of intricate causes. Furthermore, there isn't a simple, universal answer.

• Let people hear you. Whether it was overt or more covert, discuss any weight discrimination you experienced in the medical setting with your healthcare practitioner during your appointment. Notify the OAC of any instances of weight bias you witness on TV or social media so their task force can take appropriate action.

• Consult with your elected officials. Write or email a letter to the legislator representing your town or state. Encourage them to propose or back legislation that outlaws discrimination based on weight.

• Seek assistance. Participate in weight-shaming and obesity support groups, or talk to a close friend or family member about how you're feeling. To learn how to break free from self-defeating ideas that trap you in a negative cycle, think about talking to a therapist.

Being your advocate is crucial above all else. Don't be scared to "rock the boat" and practice speaking out for what you need. Like everyone else, you have a right to the same amenities and comforts. Ask your healthcare provider to supply a larger size if, for example, the patient gowns in their office are too small for you.

To be a self-advocate, you should also question your doctor about all of your alternatives for losing weight and reducing your chance of developing chronic illness. A wide range of therapies are available, such as anti-obesity drugs, bariatric surgery, and lifestyle modifications. A healthy weight can be attained and maintained by following good lifestyle practices rather than fad diets, according to public health and awareness campaigns.

Conclusion

Steer clear of risky supplements and crash diets if you want to decrease body fat sustainably.

Instead, make healthy behaviors a part of your daily routine, including drinking coffee, and probiotics, switching to sugar-free drinks, eating whole grains instead of refined carbohydrates, and so on.

For long-lasting, sustainable fat-burning, combine these easy dietary guidelines with a well-balanced diet and active lifestyle.

Tracking your weight alone is not as beneficial for tracking fat loss as using a body fat scale or skinfold caliper.

Counting the inches or centimeters that you have dropped from your hips and waist, as well as observing any changes in the way that your garments fit around your waist, are two more easy methods to track your fat loss.

Given the importance of your fat-to-muscle ratio to your general health, losing weight in the form of fat rather than muscle should be your top objective.

Eating a lot of protein, exercising, and calorie-restricting moderately are ways to make fat loss your top priority.

Losing weight requires understanding how fat loss occurs. Recall that each person's path is unique. Diet, exercise, hormones, and metabolism are some of the factors that influence fat loss and success. You have a better chance of losing weight and maintaining your health for many years to come if you follow the helpful advice provided here, which includes eating well, exercising frequently, and managing stress and sleep.

It takes perseverance, hard work, and a thorough understanding of weight loss science to lose fat. Keep in mind that changes begin small when you embark on your weight loss quest. You'll reap the rewards of a healthier, more confident version of yourself if you persevere.